The Ultimate Salad Sirtfood Diet Cookbook

50 recipes for enjoying tasty and healthy salads

Anne Patel

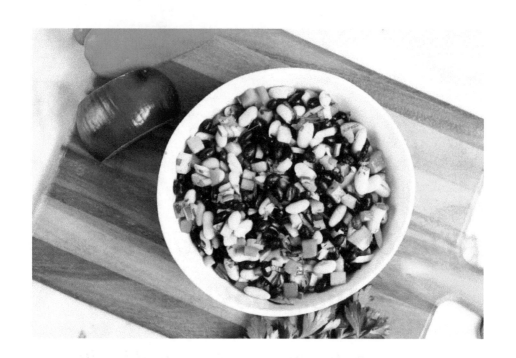

Table of Contents

Chapter 1: What is the Sirtfood diet

The Sirtfood Diet was created by Masters in Nutritional Medicine, Aiden Goggins and Glen Matten.

Their goal initially was to find a healthier way for people to eat, but people started losing weight quickly when they tested their program. With all the people in the world following diets hoping to lose pounds, they thought it would be selfish not to disclose their innovative health plan.

The plan they developed focuses on combining certain foods eaten in order to maximize the supply of nutrition to our body. There is an initial phase in which calories are limited to give the body a period to recover and eliminate accumulated waste. A maintenance phase follows this first phase to accustom the metabolism to the new foods you are ingesting. Throughout all stages, you will incorporate potent green juices and well-structured, well-planned meals.

The diet focuses on so-called 'sirtfoods,' plant-based foods that are known to stimulate a gene called sirtuin in the human body. Sirtuins belong to an entire protein family, called SIRT1 to

SIRT7, and each has specific health-related connections. These proteins help separate and safeguard our cells from inflammation and other damage resulting from everyday activities, helping to reduce our risk of developing major diseases, particularly those related to aging.

Studies have shown that people live longer and healthier lives when they eat diets rich in these foods that activate sirtuin, free from diabetes, heart disease, and even dementia. So this diet was designed to restore a healthy body situation, and one of the byproducts of a healthy body is also the loss of excess weight.

The diet Sirtfood is neither a miracle cure nor a week-long program designed to quickly lose weight before beach holidays. If you are only interested in losing a few pounds and then returning to your old habits, there are certainly plans and diets that are more suited to your needs.

The Sirtfood diet is a project born to help you for the rest of your life, using delicious foods, but that will also improve your health. If you switch from a standard American diet (SAD) to a sirtfood diet, you will lose all the weight your body does not need.

A healthy body does not store extra energy. It asks for what it needs and uses it effectively.

The diet isn't designed to encourage you to starve or deprive yourself. The fact is, foods that are deficient in nutrients are designer made to deprive you and, though the calories are there in plenty, your cells are still starved for the nutrition to help you thrive. The Sirtfood Diet is the opposite of deprivation and starvation. It is nourishment and balance.

Most people following the SAD may use 20 ingredients in a month, let alone enjoy the sheer volume of choice ingredients from the 120 options you will learn about here.

In recent decades, an alarming number of people have come to the conclusion that healthy food is boring, and plants or, more specifically, vegetables are terrible tasting. This is because the foods we've become dependent on – packed with sugar, salt, and unhealthy fats – have chemically altered our connection to food. Our brains are essentially lying to us, and our taste buds have been compromised.

This is one of the reasons the week-long reset is so important. After this first week, you will be able to taste food differently. The more you expose yourself to the recommended plant-based foods, the more pleasure you get out of them.

Sirtuins are critical for our health, regulating many essential biological functions, including our metabolism, which, I'm sure you know, is very closely connected to our weight. It's also a key figure in determining our body composition, such as how much muscle we build and how much fat we retain.

Sirtuin genes regulate all this and more. They're also integral in the process of aging and disease.

If we can turn these genes on, we'll be able to protect our cells and enjoy better health for longer life. Eating sirtfoods is the most effective way to accomplish this goal.

Sirtfoods are all plant-based, and they have many more benefits, in addition to being sirtuin activators.

Our bodies require energy to operate, and the majority of this fuel comes from three primary macronutrients: carbohydrates, fats, and proteins. These macros largely control our metabolic system and regulate how the calories we consume get processed by our bodies. This is why most diets focus exclusively on micronutrition and require you to calculate calories.

Our bodies need more than just energy to survive than thriving, however, which is why micronutrients are so important. They don't impact our weight as obviously as macros, but they are our health foundations.

Micronutrients, such as vitamins, minerals, fiber, antioxidants, and phytonutrients, are supposed to be consumed along with our calories. Unfortunately, in the Standard American Diet (SAD), they're in very limited supply.

When your diet is primarily made up of large quantities of red meat and processed meats, pre-packaged foods, vegetable oils, refined grains and a lot of sugar, you will have an almost total lack of micronutrition.

Plant foods offer the most micronutrients per calorie consumed. Every edible plant has a unique nutritional profile, protecting you from an innumerable variety of illnesses.

Sirtfoods, and other plant-based sources of nutrition, give your body what it needs to stay young and disease-free, and, as a bonus, this will help you remain at an ideal weight.

The original Sirtfood Diet encourages you to commit to a one week reset phase and then a 2-week maintenance phase where you rely heavily on the Sirtfood green juice for a significant dose of nutrition along with meals rich in sirtfoods. Once the phases are complete, to retain your health for the rest of your life, you will need to continue incorporating these sirtfoods into your daily meals.

The Sirtfood Diet is not a miracle cure, but if you stick to these recipes, you'll not just impress your taste buds, but you'll also enhance nearly every aspect of your health. To get safe, you don't have to count calories or starve yourself, the youthful body you've always wanted.

Sirtfood Diet Phases

Every newbie needs to understand that the sirtfood diet does not start with a single list of ingredients in your hands. Its implementation and adaptation are more than mere selective grocery shopping. Every diet can only work effectively when we allow our body to embrace the sudden shift and change in food intake. Similarly, the sirtfood diet also comes with two phases of adaptation. If a dieter successfully goes through these phases, he can continue with the sirtfood diet easily. There are mainly two phases of this diet, which are then succeeded by a third phase in which you can decide how you want to continue the diet.

<u>Phase One</u>

The first seven days of this diet plan are characterized as Phase One. In this phase, a dieter must focus on calorie restriction and the intake of green juices. These seven days are crucial to initiate your weight loss and usually help to lose up to seven pounds if the diet is followed properly. If you find yourself achieving this target, that means that you are on the right track.

In the first three days of the first phase, a dieter must restrict this caloric intake to 1,000 calories only. While doing so, the dieter must also have green juice throughout the day, probably three times a day. Try to drink green juice per meal. The recipes given in the book are perfect for selecting from.

Many meal options can keep your caloric intake in checks, such as buckwheat noodles, seared tofu, some shrimp stir fry, or sirtfood omelet.

Once the first three days of this diet has passed, you can increase your caloric intake to 1,500 calories per day. In these next four days, you can reduce the green juices to two times per side. And pair the juices with more Sirtuin-rich food in every meal.

Phase Two

After the first week of the sirtfood diet, then starts phase two. This phase is more about the maintenance of the diet, as the first week enables the body to embrace the change and start working according to the new diet. This phase enables the body to continue working towards the weight loss objective slowly and steadily. Therefore, the duration of this phase is almost two weeks.

So how is this phase different from phase one? In this phase, there is no restriction on the caloric intake, as long as the food is rich in sirtuins and you are taking it three times a day, it is good to go. Instead of having the green juice two or three times a day, the dieter can have juice one time a day, and that will be enough to achieve steady weight loss. You can have the juice after any meal, in the morning or in the evening.

After the Diet Phase

With the end of phase two comes the time, which is most crucial, and that is the after-diet phase. If your weight loss target has not been reached by the end of step two, then you can restart the phases all over again. Or even when you have achieved the goals but still want to lose more weight, then you can again give it a try.

Instead of following phases one and two over and over again, you can also continue having good quality sirtfood meals in this after-diet phase. Simply continue the eating practices of phase two, have a diet rich in sirtuin and do have green juices whenever possible. The diet is mainly divided into two phases: the first lasts one week, and the other lasts 14 days.

The best 20 sirt foods

All these foods include high quantities of plant compounds called polyphenols, which can be thought to modify the sirtuin enzymes, therefore, excite their super-healthy added benefits.

Top 20 sirtfoods

1. Arugula (Rocket)
2. Buckwheat
3. Capers
4. Celery
5. Chilis
6. Cocoa
7. Coffee
8. Extra Virgin Olive Oil
9. Garlic
10. Green Tea (especially Matcha)
11. Kale
12. Medjool Dates
13. Parsley
14. Red Endive
15. Red Onions
16. Red Wine
17. Soy
18. Strawberries

19. Turmeric

20. Walnuts

What Is So Great About Sirtuins?

There are seven types of Sirtuins named from **SIRT1** to **SIRT7**. Although our understanding of the exact functions of all the Sirtuins is minimal, studies show that activating them can have the following benefits:

Switching on fat burning and protection from weight gain: Sirtuins do this by increasing the mitochondrion's functionality (which is involved in the production of energy) and sparking a change in your metabolism to break down more fat cells.

Improving Memory by protecting neurons from damage. Sirtuins also boost learning skills and memory through the enhancement of synaptic plasticity. Synaptic plasticity refers to synapses' capacity to weaken or strengthen with time due to decreased or increased activity. This is important because memories are represented by different interconnected networks of synapses in the brain, and synaptic plasticity is an important neurochemical foundation of memory and learning.

Slowing down the Ageing Process: Sirtuins act as cell guarding enzymes. Thus, they protect the cells and slow down their aging process.

Repairing cells: The Sirtuins repair cells damaged by re-activating cell functionality.

Protection against diabetes: this happens through prevention against insulin resistance. Sirtuins do this by controlling blood sugar levels because this diet calls for moderate consumption of carbohydrates. These foods cause increases in blood sugar levels; hence the need to release insulin, and as the blood sugar levels increase greatly, there is a need to produce more insulin. Over time, cells become resistant to insulin, hence producing more insulin and leading to insulin resistance.

Fighting Cancers: The chemicals working as sirtuin activators affect the function of sirtuin in different cells, i.e. by switching it on when in normal cells and shutting it down in cancerous cells. This encourages the death of cancerous cells.

Fighting inflammation: Sirtuins have a powerful antioxidant effect that has the power to reduce oxidative stress. This has positive effects on heart health and cardiovascular protection.

Chapter 2: How do the Sirtfood Diet Works?

The basis of the sirtuin diet can be explained in simple terms or in complex ways. However, it's important to understand how and why it works so that you can appreciate the value of what you are doing. It is important to also know why these sirtuin rich foods help to help you maintain fidelity to your diet plan. Otherwise, you may throw something in your meal with less nutrition that would defeat the purpose of planning for one rich in sirtuins. Most importantly, this is not a dietary fad, and as you will see, there is much wisdom contained in how humans have used natural foods, even for medicinal purposes, over thousands of years.

To understand how the Sirtfood diet works and why these particular foods are necessary, we're going to look at their role in the human body.

Sirtuin activity was first researched in yeast, where a mutation caused an extension in the yeast's lifespan. Sirtuins were also shown to slow aging in laboratory mice, fruit flies, and nematodes. As research on Sirtuins proved to transfer to mammals, they were examined for their use in diet and slowing the aging process. The sirtuins in humans are different in typing, but they essentially work in the same ways and reasons.

The Sirtuin family is made up of seven "members." It is believed that sirtuins play a big role in regulating certain functions of cells, including proliferation, reproduction and growth of cells), apoptosis death of cells). They promote survival and resist stress to increase longevity.

They are also seen to block neurodegeneration loss or function of the nerve cells in the brain). They conduct their housekeeping functions by cleaning out toxic proteins and supporting the brain's ability to change and adapt to different conditions or to recuperate i.e., brain plasticity). They also help minimize chronic inflammation as part of this and decrease anything called oxidative stress. Oxidative stress is when there are so many free radicals present in the body that are cell-damaging, and by fighting them with antioxidants, the body can not keep up. These factors are related to age-related illness and weight as well, which again brings us back to a discussion of how they actually work.

You will see labels in Sirtuins that start with "SIR," which represents "Silence Information Regulator" genes. They do exactly that, silence or regulate, as part of their functions. Humans work with the seven sirtuins: SIRT1, SIRT2, SIRT3,

SIRT4, SIRT 5, SIRT6 and SIRT7. Each of these types is responsible for different areas of protecting cells. They work by either stimulating or turning on certain gene expressions or by reducing and turning off other gene expressions. This essentially means that they can influence genes to do more or less of something, most of which they are already programmed to do.

Through enzyme reactions, each of the SIRT types affects different areas of cells responsible for the metabolic processes that help maintain life. This is also related to what organs and functions they will affect.

For example, the SIRT6 causes and expression of genes in humans that affect skeletal muscle, fat tissue, brain, and heart. SIRT 3 would cause an expression of genes that affect the kidneys, liver, brain and heart.

If we tie these concepts together, you can see that the Sirtuin proteins can change the expression of genes, and in the case of the Sirtfood diet, we care about how sirtuins can turn off those genes that are responsible for speeding up aging and for weight management.

The other aspect to this conversation of sirtuins is the function and the power of calorie restriction on the human body. Calorie restriction is simply eating fewer calories. This, coupled with exercise and reducing stress, is usually a combination for weight loss. Calorie restriction has also proven across much research in animals and humans to increase one's lifespan.

We can look further at the role of sirtuins with calorie restriction and using the SIRT3 protein, which has a role in metabolism and aging. Amongst all of the effects of the protein on gene expression, such as preventing cells from dying, reducing tumors from growing, etc.), we want to understand the effects of SIRT3 on weight for this book's purpose.

As we stated earlier, the SIRT3 has high expression in those metabolically active tissues, and its ability to express itself increases with caloric restriction, fasting, and exercise. On the contrary, it will express itself less when the body has high fat, high calorie-riddled diet.

The last few highlights of sirtuins are their role in regulating telomeres and reducing inflammation, which also helps with staving off disease and aging.
Telomeres are sequences of proteins at the ends of chromosomes. When cells divide, these get shorter. As we age, they get shorter, and other stressors to the body also will contribute to this. Maintaining these longer telomeres is the key to slower aging. In addition, proper diet, along with exercise and other variables, can lengthen telomeres. SIRT6 is one of the

sirtuins that, if activated, can help with DNA damage, inflammation and oxidative stress. SIRT1 also helps with inflammatory response cycles that are related to many age-related diseases.

Calories restriction can extend life to some degree. Since this and fasting are a stressor, these factors will stimulate the SIRT3 proteins to kick in and protect the body from the stressors and excess free radicals. Again, the telomere length is affected as well.

Having laid this all out before you, you should appreciate how and why these miraculous compounds work in your favor, keep you youthful, healthy, and lean If they are working hard for you, don't you feel that you should do something too?

50 Best Salads Recipes

1. Spring Strawberry Kale Salad

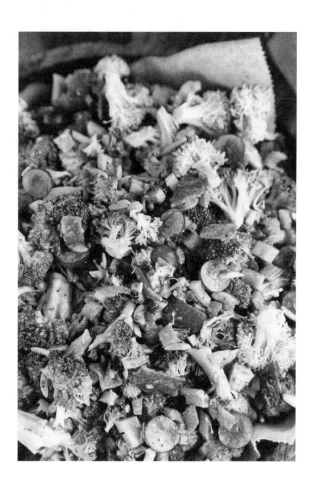

Preparation Time: 5 minutes

Cooking Time: 15-20 minutes

Servings: 4

Ingredients

3 cups baby kale, rinsed and dried

10 large strawberries, sliced

½ cup honey

1/3 cup white wine vinegar

1 cup extra virgin olive oil

1 tablespoon poppy seeds

2 tablespoons pine nuts, toasted

Salt and pepper to taste

Directions:

1. Blend the baby kale with the strawberries in a big tub.

2. To make the dressing: In a blender, add the honey, vinegar, and oil and blend until smooth.

3. Stir in the seeds of the poppy and season to taste

4. Pour over the kale and strawberries and toss to coat.

Nutrition: Calories: 220cal Carbohydrates: 21g Fat: 15g Protein: 5g

2. Blackberry Arugula Salad

Preparation Time: 5 minutes
Cooking Time: 10 minutes
Servings: 5

Ingredients

3 cups baby arugula, rinsed and dried

1-pint fresh blackberries

¾ cups of crumbled feta cheese

1-pint cherry tomatoes, halved

1 green onion, sliced

¼ cup walnuts, chopped (optional)

To Serve:

Balsamic reduction, as required

Directions:

1. In a large bowl, toss together baby arugula, blackberries, feta cheese, cherry tomatoes, green onion, and walnuts.

2. Drizzle balsamic reduction over plated salads

Nutrition: Calories: 270 Fat: 13g Saturated Fat: 2g Carbohydrates: 38g

3. Apple Walnut Spinach Salad

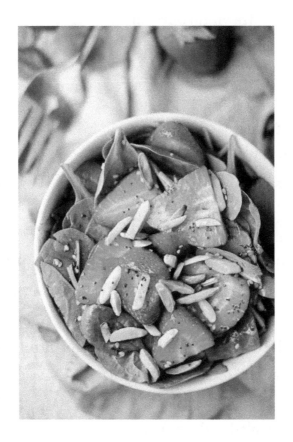

Preparation Time: 5 minutes

Cooking Time: 10 minutes

Servings: 4

Ingredients

3 cups baby spinach

1 medium apple, chopped

¼ Medjool dates, chopped

¼ cup walnuts, chopped

2 tablespoons extra virgin olive oil

1 tablespoon sugar

1 tablespoon apple cider vinegar

½ teaspoon curry powder

¼ teaspoon turmeric

1/8 teaspoon chili pepper flakes

¼ teaspoon salt

Directions:

1. Combine the spinach, apple, dates, and the walnuts in a wide bowl.

2. To make the dressing: In a jar with a tight-fitting lid, combine the remaining ingredients; shake well.

3. Drizzle over salad and toss to coat.

Nutrition: Calories: 166.1 Fat: 11.9g Cholesterol: 5.0g Carbohydrates: 12.6g

4. Enhanced Waldorf salad

Preparation Time: 5 minutes
Cooking Time: 2 hours
Servings: 4

Ingredients

4 – 5 stalks celery, sliced

1 medium apple, chopped

¼ cup walnuts, chopped

1 small red onion, diced

1 head of red endive, chopped

2 teaspoons fresh parsley, finely diced

1 tablespoon capers, drained

2 teaspoons Lovage or celery leaves, finely diced

For the dressing:

1 tablespoon extra-virgin olive oil

1 teaspoon balsamic vinegar

1 teaspoon Dijon mustard

Juice of half a lemon

Directions:

1. Whisk the milk, vinegar, mustard, and lemon juice together to make the dressing.

2. To a medium, large-sized salad bowl, add the remaining salad ingredients and toss.

3. Drizzle over the salad with the sauce, blend and serve cold.

Nutrition: Calorie: 582Kcal Fat: 103g Fat: 22.2g Protein: 8.2g

5 Kale Salad with Pepper Jelly Dressing

Preparation Time: 5 minutes - **Cooking Time:** 20 minutes - **Servings:** 4

Ingredients

4 tablespoons mild pepper jelly

3 tablespoons olive oil

¼ teaspoon salt

½ teaspoon Dijon mustard

3 cups baby kale leaves

½ cup goat cheese, crumbled

¼ cup walnuts, chopped

Directions:

1. To make the dressing: whisk the pepper jelly, olive oil, salt and mustard together in a small cup.

2. Heat in the microwave for 30 seconds. Let cool.

3. In a wide bowl, put the kale and toss with the dressing. Serve topped with goat cheese and sprinkle with walnuts.

Nutrition: Calories: 1506.3 Kcal Cholesterol: 25.3mg Carbohydrates: 96.3g

6. Hot Arugula and Artichoke Salad

Preparation Time: 5 minutes - **Cooking time**: 10 minutes - **Servings:** 2

Ingredients

1 tablespoon extra-virgin olive oil

2 cups baby arugula, washed and dried

1 red onion, thinly sliced

1 (3/4 cups) jar marinated artichoke hearts, quartered or chopped

1 cup feta cheese, crumbled

Directions:

1. Preheat oven to 300 degrees F.

2. Drizzle olive oil on a rimmed baking sheet. Spread arugula in a thick layer covering the baking sheet.

3. Arrange onions and artichokes over the spinach and drizzle the marinade from the jar over the entire salad.

4. Sprinkle with the cheese and bake until the arugula is wilted but NOT dry, or about 10 minutes.

Nutrition: Cal.: 281Kcal Fat: 26g Cholesterol:126mg Protein:7g

7. Spinach and Chicken Salad

Preparation Time: 5 minutes
Cooking Time: 30 minutes
Servings: 4

Ingredients

2 cups of rinsed and dried fresh spinach

4 cooked halves of skinless, boneless chicken breast, sliced

1 zucchini, cut lengthwise in half and sliced

1 bell pepper red, chopped

1⁄2 cup of olives in black

1⁄4 cup capers, drained

1⁄2 cups fontina cheese, frozen and shredded

Directions:

1. On four salad plates, placed equal amounts of spinach.

2. Over spinach, arrange chicken, zucchini, bell pepper, and black olives and capers and top with spinach.

3. Cheese.

Nutrition: Calories: 120   Fat: 4.9g   Cholesterol: 15mg
Carbohydrates: 13g

8. Warm Citrus Chicken Salad

Preparation Time: 10 minutes
Cooking Time: 20 minutes
Servings: 4

Ingredients

3 cups torn fresh kale

2 mandarin oranges, peeled and pulled into individual segments

½ cup mushrooms, sliced

1 small red onion, sliced

½ pound skinless, boneless chicken breast halves - cut into strips ¼ cup walnuts, chopped

2 tablespoons extra virgin olive oil

2 teaspoons cornstarch

½ teaspoon ground ginger

¼ cup pure orange juice, fresh squeezed is best ¼ cup red wine vinegar or apple cider vinegar

Directions:

1. The place was torn kale, orange segments, mushrooms, and onion into a large bowl and toss to combine.

2. In a skillet, sauté chicken and walnuts in oil stirring frequently until chicken is no longer pink, a minimum of 10 minutes.

3. In a small bowl, whisk the cornstarch, ginger, orange juice, and vinegar until smooth.

4. Stir into the chicken mixture. Bring to a boil and simmer, continually stirring for 2 minutes or until thickened and bubbly.

5. Serve salads and pour chicken mixture over the top.

Nutrition: Calories: 237
Fat: 11.3g Carbohydrates: 9.8g
Cholesterol: 101.9mg

9. Summer Buckwheat Salad

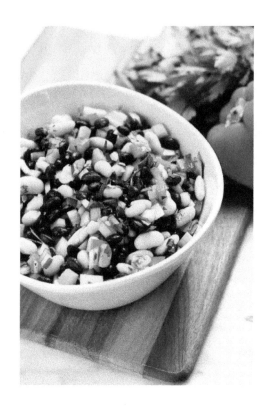

Preparation Time: 15 minutes

Cooking time: 30 minutes

Servings: 4

Ingredients

½ cup buckwheat groats

¾ cup corn kernels

2 medium-sized carrots, diced

1 spring onion, diced

¼ cucumber, chopped

1 red onion, diced

10 radishes, chopped

3 cups cooked black beans

Directions:

1. Using a fine-mesh sieve, rinse the buckwheat under running water

2. Bring to a boil in 1 cup of water, and then reduce to a simmer, covered, for 10 minutes

3. Drain well and chill in the fridge for at least 30 minutes

4. Combine cooled buckwheat and remaining ingredients in a large salad bowl

Nutrition: Calories: 128 Fat: 22g Protein: 4g

10. Greek-Style Shrimp Salad on a Bed of Baby Kale

Preparation Time: 15 minutes

Cooking Time: 30 minutes

Servings: 4

Ingredients

1-pound raw shrimp (26 to 30), peeled

¼ cup extra virgin olive oil plus more, as needed for grilling

Salt and pepper to taste

Sugar to taste

2 medium tomatoes, diced

½ cup feta cheese, crumbled

½ cup black olives, sliced

1 teaspoon dried oregano

4 teaspoons red wine vinegar

3 cups of baby kale

Directions:

1. Preheat a gas grill or barbeque on high.

2. Thread onto metal skewers with shrimp (or bamboo ones that have been soaked in water for 15 minutes).

3. Brush on both sides with oil, and season with salt, pepper, and sugar to taste.

4. Grill shrimp until spotty brown and fully cooked, about 2 minutes on each side.

5. Meanwhile, mix the tomatoes in a medium-sized dish,cheese, olives, oregano, 2 tablespoons. 2 teaspoons of vinegar and olive oil.

6. When the shrimp is cooked, unthread it carefully and add to bowl. Lightly toss all the ingredients to coat. Set aside.

7. When ready to serve, drizzle remaining oil over kale in a large bowl, tossing to coat. Add remaining vinegar and toss again.

8. Divide kale among 4 large plates. Top each of the shrimp mixture with a slice.

Nutrition: Calories: 460 Carbohydrates: 13g Fat: 33g Protein: 30g

11. Walnut Herb Pesto

Preparation Time: 5 minutes - **Cooking Time:** 3 Minutes - **Servings:** 4-6

Ingredients

1 cup walnuts

¾ cup parsley, chopped

¾ cup Lovage, chopped

¾ cup basil, chopped

½ cup Parmesan, grated

3 cloves of garlic, chopped

½ teaspoon salt

½ cup extra virgin olive oil

Directions:

1. Mix all ingredients except olive oil in a food processor and pump for a couple of seconds to combine. To get the mixture well pureed, you might need to scrape down the sides a few times.

2. Drizzle in the olive oil while the system is running to integrate the oil-once the oil is added, do not over the operation, 30 seconds is enough. Serve with crisped baguette slices or pasta

Nutrition: Calories: 31 Fat: 3.1g Carbohydrates: 0.8g

12. Creamy Lovage Dressing

Preparation Time: 5 minutes - **Cooking Time:** 0 mins - **Servings**: 2-3

Ingredients

1 lemon, juiced

1 teaspoon garlic powder

1 teaspoon dried onion powder

1 teaspoon Dijon mustard

1 teaspoon Lovage

¼ cup walnuts, soaked

1 teaspoon date or maple syrup

Salt and pepper to taste

Directions:

1. Blend the soaked nuts with the date syrup to make walnut butter.

2. Place all ingredients in a small mixing bowl.

3. Whisk well to combine.

Nutrition: Calories: 90Kcal Carbohydrates: 6g Fat: 8g Protein:0

13. Sesame Tofu Salad

Preparation Time: 12 minutes
Cooking Time: 30 minutes
Servings: 2

Ingredients

Cooked tofu – 0.625g (shredded)

Cucumber – 1 (peel, halve lengthways, deseed with a teaspoon and slice)

Sesame seeds - 1 tablespoon

Baby kale - 0.4375 g (roughly chopped)

Red onion – ½ (shredded finely)

Pak choi – ½ cup (shredded finely)

Large handful (20g) parsley, chopped

For the Dressing

Soy sauce - 2 teaspoon

Sesame oil - 1 teaspoon

Extra virgin olive oil - 1 tablespoon

Juice of 1 lime

Honey or maple syrup- 1 teaspoon

Directions:

1. Sesame seeds are toasted in a dry frying pan for approx. Two minutes, until perfumed and lightly browned. To cool, pass the seeds onto a plate.

2. Mix the lime juice, soy sauce, honey, sesame oil, and olive oil in a small bowl to get your dressing.

3. Place the Pak choi, parsley, red onion, kale, and cucumber in a large bowl. Mix. Add to the bowl of the dressing and mix again.

4. Share the salad into two plates, and then add the shredded tofu on top. Sprinkle over the sesame seeds before you serve.

Nutrition: Total Fat: 200 Carbohydrate: 8g Fat: 12g Protein: 20g

14. Turmeric Extract Poultry & Kale Salad with Honey Lime Dressing

Preparation Time: 10 minutes

Cooking time: 30 minutes

Servings: 2

Ingredients:

For the chicken:

1 teaspoon coconut oil

1/2 tool brown onion, diced

250-300 g/ 9 oz. hens mince or diced up her thighs

1 large garlic clove, finely diced

1 tsp turmeric powder

1teaspoon lime passion

Juice of 1/2 lime

1/2 tsp salt + pepper

For the salad:

6 broccoli stalks or broccoli florets

2 tablespoons pumpkin seeds (pepitas).

3 huge kale leaves, stems eliminated and chopped.

1/2 avocado, sliced.

Handful of fresh coriander leaves, chopped.

Handful of fresh parsley leaves, sliced.

For the clothing:

3 tablespoons lime juice.

1 small garlic clove, finely grated.

3 tbsps. Extra-virgin olive oil (I made use of 1 tbsp. avocado oil and * 2 tbsps. EVO).

1 tsp raw honey.

1/2 tsp wholegrain or Dijon mustard.

1/2 teaspoon sea salt and pepper.

Directions:

1. Melt the ghee or coconut oil over medium to high heat in a small frying pan. Include the onion and sauté on medium heat for 4-5 mins, until golden. Include the hen dice as well as garlic and mix for 2-3 minutes over medium-high warm, breaking it apart.

2. Add the turmeric extract, lime enthusiasm, lime juice, salt, and pepper, and cook, frequently mixing, for a further 3-4 mins. Establish the cooked dice apart.

3. While the poultry is cooking, bring a small saucepan of water to steam. Add the broccolini and prepare for 2 mins. Wash under cold water as well as cut into 3-4 pieces each.

4. Include the pumpkin seeds to the frying pan from the poultry and toast over tool warmth for 2 mins, often mixing to avoid

burning season with a little salt. Allot. Raw pumpkin seeds are too high to make use of.

5. The area sliced Kale in a salad bowl as well as pour over the clothing. Utilizing your hands, throw as well as massage the Kale with the dress. This will undoubtedly soften the Kale, kind of like what citrus juice does to fish or beef carpaccio-- it 'cooks' it slightly.

6. Finally toss via the prepared hen, broccolini, fresh, natural herbs, pumpkin seeds, and avocado pieces.

Nutrition: Calories: 368 Carbohydrate: 30.3g Protein 6.7g Fat: 27.6g

15. Buckwheat Pasta with Chicken Kale & Miso Dressing

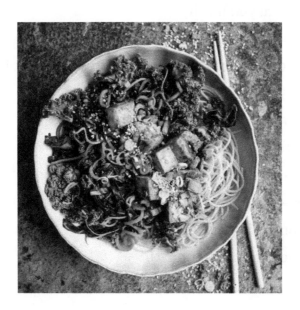

Preparation Time: 15 minutes

Cooking time: 15 minutes

Servings: 2

Ingredients:

For the noodles:

2-3 handfuls of kale leaves (eliminated from the stem as well as approximately cut).

150 g/ 5 oz. 100% buckwheat noodles.

3-4 shiitake mushrooms cut.

1 tsp coconut oil or ghee.

1 brownish onion carefully diced.

1 medium free-range chicken breast cut or diced.

1 long red chili very finely sliced (seeds in or out depending upon how warm you like it).

2 big garlic cloves finely diced.

2-3 tablespoons Tamari sauce (gluten-free soy sauce).

For the miso dressing:

1 1/2 tbsp. fresh, natural miso.

1 tbsp. Tamari sauce.

1 tbsp. extra-virgin olive oil.

1 tbsp. lemon or lime juice.

1 teaspoon sesame oil (optional).

Directions:

1. Bring a tool saucepan of water to steam. Include the Kale as well as cook for 1 min, up until a little wilted. Remove as well as reserve yet schedule the water and bring it back to the boil. Add the soba noodles and chef according to the bundle guidelines (typically about 5 mins). Rinse under cold water and allotted.

2. Then pan fry the mushrooms in coconut oil (concerning a tsp) for 2-3 minutes until gently browned on each side. Sprinkle with sea salt and allotted.

3. In the very same frypan, warmth a lot more coconut oil or ghee over medium-high warm. Sauté onion and chili for 2-3 mins and then add the poultry pieces. Cook 5 mins over medium warmth, stirring a couple of times, after that, Garlic, tamari sauce, and a small splash of water are applied. Cook for an additional 2-3 mins,, often mixing till hen is cooked via.

4. Lastly, include the kale and soba noodles and toss with the poultry to warm up.

5. Mix the dressing and drizzle over the noodles right at the end of cooking; this way, you will certainly maintain all those beneficial probiotics in the miso to life as well as energetic.

Nutrition: Calories: 260 Carbohydrate: 35.3g Protein 15g Cholesterol: 50g Fat: 27.6g

16. Sirtfood Lentil Super Salad

Preparation Time: 10 minutes
Cooking time: 0 minutes
Servings: 1

Ingredients:

20 g red onion, sliced

1 tbsp. extra virgin olive oil

1 large Medjool date, chopped

1 tbsp. capers

¼ cup rocket

2 avocados, peeled, stoned and sliced

100 g lentils

¼ cup chicory leaves

2 tbsp. chopped walnuts

1 tbsp. fresh lemon juice

¼ cup chopped parsley

¼ cup chopped celery leaves

Directions:

1. Arrange salad leaves in a large bowl or a plate; mix the remaining ingredients well and serve over the salad leaves.

Nutrition: Calories: 456 Carbs: 54 Protein: 27 Fat: 11

17. Sirty Fruit Salad

Preparation Time: 10 minutes
Cooking time: 0 minutes
Servings: 1

Ingredients:

10 blueberries

10 red seedless grapes

½ cup brewed green tea

1 apple, cored, chopped

1 tsp. honey

1 orange, chopped

2 tbsp. fresh lemon juice

Directions:

1. Add honey into a cup of green tea and stir until dissolved; add orange juice and set aside to cool.

2. Place the chopped orange in a bowl and add grapes, apple and blueberries; Pour over the tea and leave to steep before serving for at least 5 minutes.

Nutrition: Calories per serving: 362.47 kcal Carbs per serving: 25.39 g Fats per serving: 9.34 g Proteins per serving: 5.28 g Fiber per serving: 2.86 g Sodium per serving: 9.

18. Superfood Cleansing Salad with Citrus Dressing

Preparation Time: 15 minutes
Cooking time: 0 minutes
Servings: 4

Ingredients:

2 cups red cabbage, chopped

2 cups kale, chopped

1 head cauliflower, roughly chopped

1 red onion

2 cups baby carrots

1/3 cup fresh cilantro, chopped

1/3 cup sunflower seeds

1/2 cup raisins

1/2 cup raw hemp hearts Citrus Dressing:

2 tablespoons fresh lime juice

2 tablespoons fresh lemon juice

1/3 cup apple cider vinegar

1/2 avocado

2 cloves garlic

1/2 tablespoon fresh cilantro

1/2 tablespoon minced ginger

1/2 tablespoon raw honey

1/2 teaspoon sea salt

1/4 teaspoon pepper

Directions

1. Combine cabbage, kale, cauliflower, onion, carrots and cilantro in a food processor; shred.

2. Transfer the shredded veggies to a large bowl and fold in sunflower seeds, hemp hearts and raisins.

3. In a blender, mix all of the dressing ingredients and blend until very smooth.

4. Serve the salad in salad bowls drizzled with the citrus dressing. Enjoy!

Nutrition: Calories 91 kcal Fat 8.3 g Cholesterol 0 mg Carbohydrate 12.5 g Fat 0.5 g Protein 4. 4 g Sodium 810 mg

19. Sweet & Sour Bean Curry Salad

Preparation Time: 15 minutes
Cooking time: 40 minutes
Servings: 4

Ingredients:

½ cup garbanzo beans, rinsed, drained

1 teaspoon extra virgin olive oil

1/8 teaspoon sea salt

2 teaspoons sunflower oil

2 teaspoons freshly squeezed lemon juice

½ teaspoon lemon zest

½ teaspoon raw honey

A pinch of black pepper

¼ cup chopped bird eye's chili pepper

1 peeled mandarin orange, chopped

½ cup chopped purple cabbage

½ cup cooked quinoa

1 tablespoon toasted walnuts

Directions

1. On a baking sheet, spread the beans and bake at 450 °F for about 30 minutes or until lightly browned and slightly crunchy. Remove the beans from oven and let cool completely.

2. Toss together the baked beans, oil, and salt and return to oven for 10 more minutes or until crispy and browned. Remove from oven and let cool.

3. Whisk the sunflower oil, lemon juice, zest, sugar, sea salt and black pepper together in a bowl; set aside.

4. In a bowl, toss together the roasted beans with chopped mandarin orange, bird's eye chili pepper, cabbage and cooked quinoa; drizzle with the dressing and sprinkle with toasted walnuts to serve.

Nutrition: Calories: 534 calories Fat: 6 g Sodium: 693 mg Carbohydrates: 89.7 g Fiber: 2.1 g Sugar: 53 g Protein: 20. 2 g

20. Strawberry & Cucumber Salad

Preparation Time: 10 minutes- **Cooking time:** 0 minutes - **Servings**: 1

Ingredients:

8 strawberries, sliced

1 cucumber, sliced

Pinch of sea salt

Pinch of white pepper

Stevia

Dressing:

4 tablespoons fresh lemon juice

1 tablespoon extra-virgin olive oil

1 tablespoon apple cider vinegar

½ cup chopped strawberries

Pinch of salt

Pinch of pepper

Directions

1. Mix the salad ingredients in a big tub, in a blender, blend together dressing ingredients until smooth and pour over the salad. Toss to coat well and serve.

Nutrition: Calories - 8 (700 kg.), P - 0.24 g, F - 0.02 g, C - 0. 58 g, Sodium - 0.30 e%, Omega-6 - 0.02 g, Omega-3 - 0.05 g.

21. Sweet Kale & Cranberry Salad

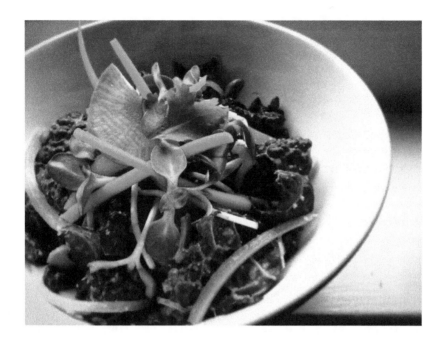

Preparation Time: 20 minutes

Cooking time: 0 minutes

Servings: 6

Ingredients:

2 large peeled sweet potatoes, cubed

2 bunches kale, chopped into small pieces

1 tablespoon fresh lemon juice

3 tablespoons extra-virgin olive oil

1/4 cup Sunflower seeds

½ cup toasted walnuts, chopped

1/2 cup dried cranberries

1 teaspoon Dijon mustard

A pinch of sea salt

A pinch of freshly ground pepper

Directions

1. In a medium saucepan, put the potatoes and cover with water; stir in a pinch of salt and bring to a gentle boil. Simmer and simmer for about 15 minutes or until the potatoes are soft; drain and cool for about 15 minutes.

2. Whisk the mustard, lemon juice and extra virgin olive oil together in a large cup.

3. Add the sweet potatoes along with all the remaining ingredients; toss to mix well and serve.

Nutrition: 25 grams of sugar, 225 calories

22. Super Raw Power Salad

Preparation Time: 10 minutes
Cooking time: 0 minutes
Servings: 8

Ingredients:
For the Dressing:
¼ cup white apple cider vinegar
¾ cup extra virgin olive oil
1 tablespoon raw honey
1/8 teaspoon garlic powder
1/8 teaspoon sea salt
2 apples, finely chopped
½ cup bean sprouts
½ cup frozen edamame, thawed
¾ cup dried berries
1½ cups chopped purple cabbage
4 cups finely chopped kale
½ cup raw sunflower seeds
Pinch of sea salt
Pinch of pepper

Directions:
1. In a sealable jar, mix all dressing ingredients and shake until well blended.

2. In a large bowl, mix all salad ingredients; pour about ¼ cup of the dressing over the salad and toss to coat well. Season with salt and pepper and serve.

Nutrition: 426 calories, 6g protein, 94g carbs, 18g fat, 171mg sodium

23. Apple, Carrot, Cucumber & Mixed Greens Salad w/ Raspberry Vinaigrette

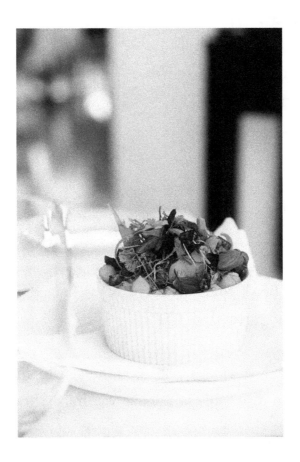

Preparation Time: 10 minutes

Cooking time: 0 minutes

Servings: 1

Ingredients:

1 cup microgreens

1/2-pound mixed greens

1/2 tart apple, chopped

1/2 small cucumber, thinly sliced

3 carrots, sliced

1 tablespoon sherry vinegar

2 tablespoons extra virgin olive oil

1 tablespoons mustard

Handful of blueberries

Pinch of sea salt

Pinch of pepper

1 hardboiled egg, chopped

Directions:

1. In a large bowl, combine microgreens, mixed greens, apple, cucumber, and carrots.

2. Combine sherry vinegar, olive oil, mustard, blueberries, salt and pepper in a sealable jar; shake vigorously to combine well and pour over the salad. Serve on plates topped with chopped hardboiled egg.

Nutrition: Calories: 177 Total fat: 22 g Saturated fat: 3.9 g Carbohydrates:14.3 g Sugar: 11.2 g Fiber: 5.2 g Protein: 3.2 g Sodium: 123 mg

24. Sirtfood Salad with Citrus Dressing

Preparation Time: 25 minutes
Cooking time: 0 minutes
Servings: 6

Ingredients:

For salad

2 cup red cabbage, finely sliced

2 cup kale, finely sliced

1 cup parsley, chopped

1 bird eye's chili, diced

1 cup radish, sliced in matchsticks

2 cup broccoli, chopped in ¼-inch pieces

1 cup carrot, sliced in matchsticks

1 cup raw walnuts, chopped

2 avocados, peeled and diced

2 tablespoons sesame seeds

freshly ground black pepper to taste

½ cup fresh lemon juice

½ cup fresh orange juice

½ cup extra-virgin olive oil

1 teaspoon minced ginger

1 tablespoon raw honey

Pinch of cayenne

¼ teaspoon sea salt

Directions:

1. Process dressing ingredients until very smooth.

2. Combine salad ingredients in a salad bowl; pour the dressing over the salad and toss to combine well. Enjoy!

Nutrition: carb: 37.9g, fat: 14.8g, protein: 57.

25. Kale Avocado Salad with Orange

Preparation Time: 10 minutes
Cooking time: 0 minutes
Servings: 2

Ingredients:

Salad

2-3 handfuls kale, rinsed and chopped

½ cup green peas

½ avocado, sliced

½ cucumber, sliced

1 orange, sliced

2 tablespoons chopped toasted walnut

2 tablespoons hemp seeds, shelled Vinaigrette

2 tablespoons extra virgin olive oil

3 tablespoons lemon juice

Pinch garlic powder

Sea salt

Black pepper

Directions

1. In a saucepan, place the chopped kale. In a small bowl, mix extra virgin olive oil, lemon juice, garlic powder, sea salt and pepper; rub the lemon vinaigrette with your hands into the kale for approximately 2 minutes or until the kale begins to soften.

2. Divide the between two serving plates and add peas, avocado, cucumber, and orange slices.

3. Top with almond slices and hemp seeds; drizzle with lemon juice and sprinkle with cracked pepper. Enjoy!

Nutrition: Calories: 80g Total fat: 6.6g Protein: 1.6g Carbohydrate: 1. 5g Sugar: 0.3g Sodium: 0. 5g

26. Caesar Dressing

Preparation Time: 10 minutes
Cooking Time: 5 minutes
Servings: 1 cup

Ingredients:

250 ml Olive oil

2 tablespoons Lemon juice

4 pieces Anchovy fillet

2 tablespoon Mustard yellow

1 clove Garlic

½ teaspoon Salt

½ teaspoon Black pepper

Directions:

1. Remove the garlic peel and finely chop it.

2. Put all ingredients in a blender and puree evenly.

3. It is possible to keep this dressing for about 3 days in the fridge.

Nutrition: Calories: 71 Cal Fat: 2.78 g Carbs: 6.76 g Protein: 6.38 g Fiber: 2.1 g

27. Basil Dressing

Preparation Time: 10 minutes - **Cooking Time:** 5 minutes - **Servings:** 1 cup

Ingredients:

100 g fresh basil

1 pc Shallots

1 clove Garlic

125 ml Olive oil (mild)

2 tbsp White wine vinegar

Directions:

1. Finely chop the shallot and garlic.

2. Put the shallot, garlic, basil, olive oil and vinegar in a blender.

3. Mix it into an even mix.

4. Season the dressing and season with salt and pepper.

5. Place the dressing in a clean glass and store in the refrigerator. It stays fresh and tasty for at least 3 days.

Nutrition: Calories: 33 Cal Fat: 0.66 g Carbs: 3.72 g Protein: 3.35 g Fiber: 1.7 g

28. Strawberry Sauce

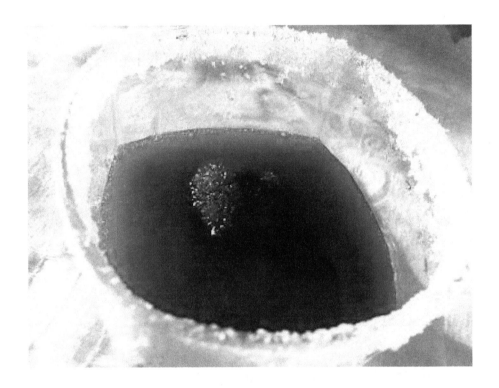

Preparation Time: 15 minutes

Cooking Time: 15 minutes

Servings: 1 cup

Ingredients:

225 g Strawberries

3 tablespoons Coconut blossom sugar

4 tablespoons Honey

125 ml Water

2 teaspoon Arrowroot powder

Directions:

1. Roughly chop strawberries.

2. Put the strawberries in a pan with coconut blossom sugar and honey. Place the pan on medium heat.

3. In the meantime, mix the arrow roots with a whisk in the water. Add this mixture to the strawberries.

4. Heat the strawberries until they start to bubble and start to thicken. (Not cook!)

5. Your strawberry sauce is ready after about 15 minutes. Store the sauce in a clean glass refrigerator.

Nutrition: Calories: 238 Cal Fat: 3.91 g Carbs: 105.68 g Protein: 2.81 g Fiber: 5.4 g

29. Fresh Chicory Salad

Preparation Time: 15 minutes - **Cooking Time:** 5 minutes - **Servings:** 2 – 3

Ingredients:

1 piece Orange

1 piece Tomato

¼ pieces Cucumber

1/4 pieces Red onion

Directions:

1. Cut off the hard stem of the chicory and remove the leaves.

2. Peel the orange and cut the pulp into wedges.

3. Break the cucumbers and tomatoes into small bits.

4. Cut the red onion into thin half rings.

5. Place the chicory boats on a plate, spread the orange wedges, tomato, cucumber and red onion over the boats.

6. Sprinkle some olive oil and fresh lemon juice on the dish.

Nutrition: Calories: 73 Cal Fat: 0.49 g Carbs: 15.73 g Protein: 2.68 g Fiber: 3.5 g

30. Grilled Vegetables And Tomatoes

Preparation Time: 10 minutes
Cooking Time: 10 minutes
Servings: 2 – 3

Ingredients:
1 piece Zucchini

1 piece Eggplant

3 pieces Tomatoes

1 piece Cucumber

Dressing:

4 tablespoons Olive oil

110 ml Orange juice (fresh)

1 tablespoon Apple cider vinegar

1 hand fresh basil

Directions:
1. Cut all of the vegetables into equally thick slices (about half a centimeter).

2. Heat the grill pan and fry the zucchini and eggplant.

3. While the zucchini and eggplant are fried, season with salt and pepper.

4. Remove the basil leaves from the branches.

5. Spread the vegetables alternately on a plate.

6. Add a leaf of basil every now and then.

7. Mix the ingredients for the dressing and serve the dressing separately on the side.

Nutrition: Calories: 168 Cal Fat: 55.53 g Carbs: 40.39 g Protein: 7.7 g Fiber: 18.7 g

31. Steak Salad

Preparation Time: 10 minutes

Cooking Time: 10 minutes

Servings: 2 – 3

Ingredients:

2 pieces Beef steak

2 cloves Garlic

1 piece Red onion

2 pieces Egg

1 hand Cherry tomatoes

2 hands Lettuce

1 piece Avocado

½ pieces Cucumber

1 pinch Season white Salt

1 pinch Black pepper

Directions:

1. Place the steaks in a flat bowl.

2. Pour the olive oil over the steaks and press the garlic over it. Turn the steaks a few times so that they are covered with oil and garlic.

3. Cover the meat and allow it to marinate for at least 1 hour.

4. Boil eggs.

5. Heat a grill pan and fry the steaks medium.

6. Take the steaks out of the pan, wrap them in aluminum foil and let them rest for 5 to 10 minutes.

7. Spread the lettuce on the plates.

8. Cut the steaks into slices and place them in the middle of the salad.

9. Cut the eggs into wedges, the cucumber into half-moons, the red onion into thin half-rings, cherry tomatoes into halves and slices of avocado.

10. Spread this around the steaks.

11. Sprinkle over the olive oil and white wine vinegar and season with a little salt and pepper.

Nutrition: Calories: 131 Cal Fat: 74.9 g Carbs: 37.09 g Protein: 23 g Fiber: 17 g

32. Zucchini Salad With Lemon Chicken

Preparation Time: 1 hour 10 minutes
Cooking Time: 25 minutes
Servings: 2 – 3

Ingredients:

1 piece Zucchini

1 piece yellow zucchini

1 hand Cherry tomatoes

2 pieces Chicken breast

1 piece Lemon

2 tablespoons Olive oil

Directions:

1. Utilize a meat mallet or a heavy pan to make the chicken fillets as thin as possible.

2. Put the fillets in a bowl.

3. Over the chicken, squeeze the lemon and apply the olive oil. Cover it and leave for at least 1 hour to marinate.

4. Heat a pan over medium-high heat and fry the chicken until cooked through and browned.

5. Season with salt and pepper.

6. Make zucchini from the zucchini and put in a bowl.

7. Quarter the tomatoes and stir in the zucchini.

8. Slice the chicken fillets diagonally and place them on the salad.

9. Drizzle a little olive oil with the salad and season with salt and pepper.

Nutrition: Calories: 125 Cal Fat: 80.83 g Carbs: 4.97 g Protein: 121.48 g Fiber: 0.4 g

33. Fresh Salad With Orange Dressing

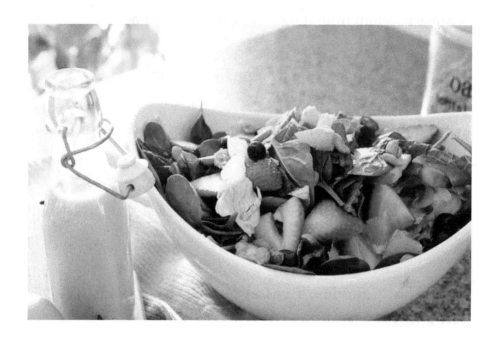

Preparation Time: 10 minutes

Cooking Time: 5 minutes

Servings: 2 – 3

Ingredients:

1 / 2 fruit Salad

1 piece yellow bell pepper

1 piece Red pepper

100 g Carrot (grated)

1 hand Almonds

Dressing:

4 tablespoon Olive oil

110 ml Orange juice (fresh)

1 tablespoon Apple cider vinegar

Directions:

1. Clean the peppers and cut them into long thin strips.

2. Tear off the lettuce leaves and cut them into smaller pieces.

3. Mix the salad with the peppers and the carrots processed with the Julienne peeler in a bowl.

4. Chop the almonds roughly and scatter over the salad.

5. In a tub, combine all the ingredients for the dressing. Just prior to eating, pour the dressing over the salad.

Nutrition: Calories: 158 Cal Fat: 55.07 g Carbs: 16.84 g Protein: 2.76 g Fiber: 4.5 g

34. Tomato And Avocado Salad

Preparation Time: 10 minutes
Cooking Time: 5 minutes
Servings: 2 – 3

Ingredients:

1 piece Tomato

1 hand Cherry tomatoes

½ pieces Red onion

1 piece Avocado

Taste fresh oregano

1 1 / 2 EL Olive oil

1 teaspoon White wine vinegar

1 pinch Celtic sea salt

Directions:

1. Cut the tomato into thick slices.

2. Cut half of the cherry tomatoes into slices and the other half in half.

3. Cut the red onion into super thin half rings. (or use a mandolin for this)

4. Cut the avocado into 6 parts.

5. Spread the tomatoes on a plate, place the avocado on top and sprinkle the red onion over them.

6. Sprinkle fresh oregano on the salad as desired.

7. Drizzle olive oil and vinegar on the salad with a pinch of salt.

Nutrition: Calories: 138 Cal Fat: 29.65 g Carbs: 29.86 g Protein: 5.6 g Fiber: 15.8 g

35. Arugula With Fruits And Nuts

Preparation Time: 10 minutes

Cooking Time: 5 minutes

Servings: 2 – 3

Ingredients:

75 g Arugula

2 pieces Peach

½ pieces Red onion

1 hand Blueberries

Pecans 1 hand

Dressing:

½ pieces Peach

65 ml Olive oil

2 tablespoon White wine vinegar

1 sprig fresh basil

1 pinch Salt

1 pinch Black pepper

Directions:

1. Halve the 2 peaches and remove the core.

2. Cut the pulp into pieces.

3. Heat a grill pan and grill the peaches briefly on both sides.

4. Cut the red onion into thin half rings.

5. Roughly chop the pecans.

6. Heat a pan and roast the pecans in it until they are fragrant.

7. Place the arugula on a plate and spread it over the peaches, red onions, blueberries and roasted pecans.

8. Place all the dressing ingredients in a blender or food processor and mix with a smooth dressing.

9. Drizzle the dressing over the salad.

Nutrition: Calories: 68 Cal Fat: 0.61 g Carbs: 13.09 g Protein: 3.16 g Fiber: 3.1 g

36. Spinach Salad With Green Asparagus And Salmon

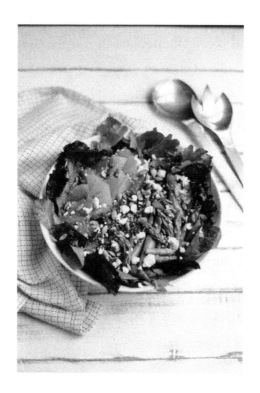

Preparation Time: 10 minutes

Cooking Time: 5 minutes

Servings: 2 – 3

Ingredients:

2 hands Spinach

2 pieces Egg

120 g smoked salmon

100 g Asparagus tips

150 g Cherry tomatoes

Lemon ½ pieces

1 teaspoon Olive oil

Directions:

1. Make the eggs the way they please you.

2. Heat a pan with a little oil and fry the asparagus tips al dente.

3. Halve cherry tomatoes.

4. Place the spinach on a plate and spread the asparagus tips, cherry tomatoes and smoked salmon on top.

5. Scare, peel and halve the eggs. Add them to the salad.

6. Squeeze the lemon over the lettuce and drizzle some olive oil over it.

7. Season the salad with a little salt and pepper.

Nutrition: Calories: 208 Cal Fat: 32.92 g Carbs: 33.24 g Protein: 46.65 g Fiber: 5.4 g

37. Brunoise Salad

Preparation Time: 10 minutes
Cooking Time: 5 minutes
Servings: 1

Ingredients:

1 piece Meat tomato

½ pieces Zucchini

½ pieces Red bell pepper

½ pieces yellow bell pepper

½ pieces Red onion

3 sprigs fresh parsley

½ pieces Lemon

2 tablespoons Olive oil

Directions:

1. Finely dice the tomatoes, zucchini, peppers and red onions to get a brunoise.

2. Mix all the cubes in a bowl.

3. Chop parsley and mix in the salad.

4. Over the salad, squeeze the lemon and apply the olive oil.

5. Season with salt and pepper.

Nutrition: Calories: 268 Cal Fat: 28.06 g Carbs: 28.39 g Protein: 5.64 g Fiber: 5.4 g

38. Broccoli Salad

Preparation Time: 10 minutes
Cooking Time: 5 minutes
Servings: 1

Ingredients:
1 piece Broccoli
½ pieces Red onion
100 g Carrot (grated)
1 hand Red grapes

Dressing:
2 ½ tablespoon Coconut yogurt
1 tablespoon Water
1 teaspoon Mustard yellow
1 pinch Salt

Directions:
1. Slice the broccoli into small florets and cook al dente for 5 minutes.

2. Cut the red onion into thin half rings.

3. Halve the grapes.

4. Mix coconut yogurt, water and mustard with a pinch of salt to make an even dressing.

5. Drain the broccoli and rinse with ice-cold water to stop the cooking process.

6. Mix the broccoli with the carrot, onion and red grapes in a bowl.

7. Serve the dressing separately on the side.

Nutrition: Calories: 91 Cal Fat: 0.52 g Carbs: 20.79 g Protein: 2.41 g Fiber: 5.4 g

39. Kale & Feta Salad

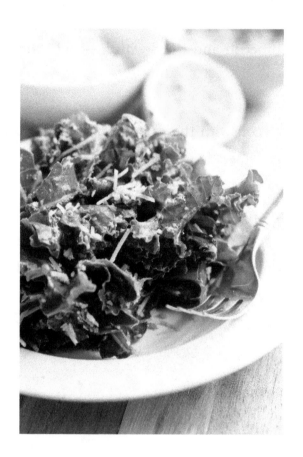

Preparation Time: 10 minutes

Cooking Time: 0 minute

Servings: 1

Ingredients:

250g kale, finely chopped

50g walnuts, chopped

75g feta cheese, broken

1 apple, peeled, cored & diced

4 medjool dates, chopped

75g cranberries

½ red onion, chopped

3 tbsp. olive oil

3 tbsp. water

2 tsp honey, 1 tbsp. red wine vinegar

A pinch of salt

Directions:

1. In a bowl, throw together the kale, walnuts, feta cheese, apple, and dates, and then stir.

2. In a food processor, add cranberries, red onion, olive oil, water, honey, red wine vinegar, and a pinch of salt. Process until smooth and fluid, adding water if necessary. Pour the cranberry dressing over the salad and serve.

Nutrition: Calories: 186 Fiber: 2.5 g

40. Crowning Celebration Chicken Salad

Preparation Time: 5 minutes - **Cooking Time:** 10 minutes - **Servings:** 1

Ingredients:

75 g Natural yogurt

Juice of 1/4 of a lemon

1 tsp Coriander, cleaved

1 tsp Ground turmeric

1/2 tsp Mild curry powder

100 g Cooked chicken bosom, cut into scaled down pieces

6 Walnut parts, finely shredded

1 Medjool date, finely shredded

20 g Red onion, diced

1 Bird's eye bean stew

40 g Rocket, to serve

Directions:

1. Blend the yogurt, lemon juice, coriander and flavors together in a bowl.

2. Attach all of the remaining ingredients and serve on the rocket bed.

Nutrition: Calories 314 Fat: 13 g Carbohydrates: 28 g Protein: 2 g Fiber: 1 g

41. Sirt Super Salad

Preparation Time: 15 Minutes - **Cooking Time:** 15 Minutes - **Servings:** 1

Ingredients:

1 ¾ ounces (50g) arugula

1 ¾ ounces (50g) endive leaves

3 ½ ounces (100g) smoked salmon cuts

½ cup (80g) avocado, stripped, stoned, and cut 1/2 cup (50g) celery including leaves, cut 1/8 cup (20g) red onion, cut 1/8 cups (15g) pecans, shredded

1 tablespoon escapades

1 enormous Medjool date, hollowed and shredded

1 tablespoon additional virgin olive oil

juice of ¼ lemon

¼ cup (10g) parsley, shredded

Directions:

1. Spot, the serving of mixed greens, leaves on a plate or in an enormous bowl.

2. Combine and serve over the leaves with all the rest of the ingredients.

Nutrition: Calories 236 Fat: 13 g Carbohydrates: 28 g Protein: 2 g

42. Walnuts Avocado Salad

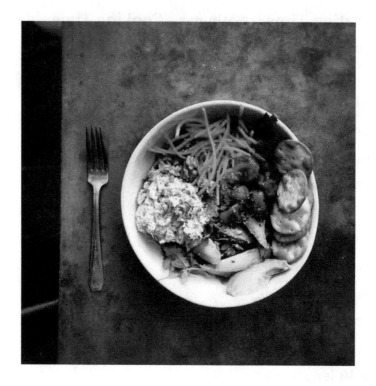

Preparation Time: 8 minutes - **Cooking Time:** 0 minutes - **Servings:** 1

Ingredients:

¼ cup of chopped parsley

¼ lemon juice

1 tbsp. of extra virgin olive oil

1 large Medjool date, pitted and chopped

1 tbsp. of capers

1/8 cups of chopped walnuts

1/8 cup of sliced red onion

½ cup of celery including leaves, sliced

½ cup of avocado, peeled, stoned, and sliced 100 grams of smoked salmon slices (3 ½ oz.)

50 grams of endive leaves (1 ¾ oz.)

50 grams of arugula (1 ¾ oz.)

Directions:

1. Place the endive leaves, parsley, celery leaves and arugula in a large bowl or plate.

2. Mix together the remaining ingredients and serve over of the leaves.

Nutrition: Calories 89 Sugar 2 Carbohydrate 33 Vitamin K and C

43. Poached Pear Salad with Dijon Vinegar Dressing

Preparation Time: 15 minutes
Cooking Time: 0 minutes
Servings: 1

Ingredients:

For The Dressing

75 ml olive oil

75 ml walnut oil

1 tbsp. of red wine vinegar

1 tbsp. of Dijon mustard

Freshly ground Pepper to taste

Salt to taste

For The Salad

200 grams of Gorgonzola cheese, slice finely Few rocket leaves

100 grams of Walnuts

2 Ripe pears (peeled and core) cut into quarters

2 Bay leaves

Small bunch of thyme

40 grams of caster sugar

180 ml of red wine

Directions:

1. Boil the wine in a saucepan. Along with the bay leaves, sugar and thyme. Simmer over medium-low heat.

2. Add the pear into the simmering liquid and poach for 10 minutes. Remove from the heat of the pan and set aside in poaching fluid to cool pears.

3. Mix the mustard, salt, vinegar, and pepper together in a bowl until well whisked; steam in the oil slowly and whisk as you apply.

4. Arrange salad ingredients on a serving plate and drizzle with the dressing.

Nutrition: Calories 88 Sugar 4 Carbohydrate 24

44. Steak Arugula Strawberry Salad

Preparation Time: 10 minutes

Cooking Time: 15 minutes

Servings: 4

Ingredients:

Steak:

1/2 tbsp. extra virgin olive oil

Montreal steak seasoning

2 Beef tenderloin steaks

Salad:

1/8 cup of slivered walnuts

1/4 cup of crumbled feta cheese

1/2 cup of sliced strawberries

1/2 cup blueberries

1/2 cup of raspberries

3 cups of arugula

Balsamic Vinaigrette

Salt and pepper

1/4 tsp of Dijon mustard

1 1/2 tsp of sugar

1/8 cup of olive oil

1/8 cup of balsamic vinegar

Directions:

1. Steak:

2. Run the Montreal steak seasoning all over the steak and let sit for 5-10 minutes.

3. Heat oil over medium high heat in a cast-iron skillet. Once it's simmering, add in the steak and cook about 5-7 minutes; flip and cook the other side for 3-4 minutes or until its cooked the way you like your meet.

4. Set steak aside in a plate and let cool for 5 minutes before slicing into strips.

5. Salad:

6. Combine together the salad ingredients in a large bowl.

7. In a small shaker, add together the all vinaigrette ingredients and shake until well mixed. Pour the dressing over the lettuce and toss to cover evenly.

8. To Serve

9. Divide the salad into 2 bowls, then cover it with the steak.

10. Notes:

11. You can keep the dressing for up to one week in the fridge.

Nutrition: kcal: 506 Net carbs: 17g Fat: 37g Fiber: 5g Protein: 23 g

45. Super Fruit Salad

Preparation Time: 10 minutes - **Cooking Time:** 0 minutes - **Servings:** 1

Ingredients:

10 blueberries

10 red seedless grapes

1 apple, cored and chopped roughly

1 orange, halved

1 tsp of honey

½ cup of freshly made matcha green tea

Directions:

1. Combine 1/2 cup green tea with the honey and stir until dissolved, Squeeze in half of the orange into the green tea mix. Leave to cool.

2. Chop the second orange half into pieces and transfer into a bowl. Add in the blueberries, chopped apple and grapes. Pour the cooled tea on top the salad mix and allow to soak a little before serving.

Nutrition: kcal: 200 Net carbs: 40g Fat: 1g Fiber: 5g Protein: 2 g

46. Sirtfood Salmon Lentils Salad

Preparation Time: 10 minutes

Cooking Time: 0 minutes

Servings: 1

Ingredients:

20 grams of sliced red onion

40 grams of sliced celery

10 grams of chopped lovage

10 grams of chopped parsley

Juice of 1/4 of a lemon

1 tbsp. of extra virgin olive oil

1 large Medjool date, remove pit and chopped

1 tbsp. of capers

15 grams of chopped walnuts

80 grams of avocado, peeled, pitted and sliced

100g tinned green lentils or cooked Puy lentils

50 grams of chicory leaves

50 grams of rocket

Directions:

1. On a large plate, add the salad leaves.

2. Mix together the remaining ingredients and spread mixture over leaves to serve.

Nutrition: kcal: 400 Net carbs: 20g Fat: 25g Fiber: 14g Protein: 10 g

47. Blueberry Kale Salad with Ginger Lime Dressing

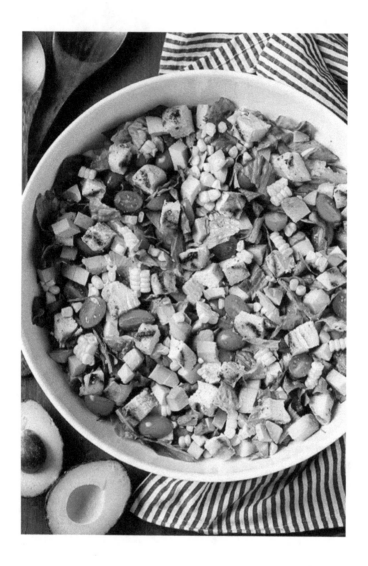

Preparation Time: 10 minutes

Cooking Time: 60 minutes

Servings: 4

Ingredients:

3 tbsps. of white wine vinegar

1 tbsp. of honey

2 tbsps. of finely chopped ginger, crystallized

3 tbsps. of lime juice

Salt and pepper to taste

Salad:

1/4 cup of slivered walnuts toasted

1/2-3/4 cup of fresh blueberries

1/3 thinly sliced red onion

8 cups of kale, de-stemmed and chopped into pieces

Directions:

1. Combine together the entire dressing ingredients in a medium bowl until well mixed.

2. Add sliced onion chopped kale, toss to coat. Leave to marinate for about 1-4 hours, depending on how much time you have, tossing periodically. This is an important step to remove the bitterness from the kale.

3. Add toasted walnuts and blueberries. Toss to coat.

Nutrition: kcal: 91 Net carbs: 10g Fat: 3.69g Fiber: 3g Protein: 3g

48. Fancy Chicken Salad

Preparation Time: 1 minute - **Cooking Time:** 10 minutes
Servings: 1

Ingredients:

1 bird's eye chili

20 grams of diced red onion

1 finely chopped medjool date

6 finely chopped Walnut halves

100 grams of cooked chicken breast, chopped into bite-sized chunks

1/2 tsp of mild curry powder

1 tsp of ground turmeric

1 tsp of chopped Coriander

Juice of 1/4 of a lemon

75 grams of natural yoghurt

40 grams of rocket

Directions:

1. Mix together the lemon juice in a tub,yoghurt, spices and coriander. Mix in the other ingredients until well blended.

2. Serve over bed of the rocket.

Nutrition: kcal: 340 Net carbs: 22g Fat: 13g Fiber: 5g Protein: 36g

49. Olive, Tomato, Yellow Pepper, Red Onion, Cucumber Slices and Feta Skewers

Preparation Time: 5 minutes
Cooking Time: 0 minutes
Servings: 2

Ingredients:
100 grams of feta, cut into 8 cubes
100 grams of cucumber, cut in quarters and halved Half red onion, cut in half and sliced into 8 pieces
1 yellow pepper (or any color you like) cut into 8 squares
8 cherry tomatoes
8 large black olives
2 wooden skewers, soaked for 30 minutes in water before use

For the dressing:
½ crushed clove garlic
1 tsp of balsamic vinegar
½ lemon Juice
Few finely chopped basil leaves (or ½ tsp of dried mixed herbs)
1 tbsp. of extra virgin olive oil
Few leaves finely chopped oregano (Skip this if using dried mixed herbs)
Freshly ground black pepper

Salt to taste

Directions:

1. Pierce each skewer through the olive, tomato, yellow pepper, red onion, cucumber slices and feta. Repeat a second time.

2. Combine the dressing ingredients in a sealable container and mix thoroughly. Pour dressing over the skewers.

Nutrition: kcal: 228 Net carbs: 13g Fat: 15g Fiber: 3g Protein: 8.7g

50. Sesame Soy Chicken Salad

Preparation Time: 10 minutes
Cooking Time: 0 minutes
Servings: 2

Ingredients:

150 grams of cooked chicken, shredded Large handful of chopped parsley (20g) ½ finely sliced red onion

60 grams of bok choy, very finely shredded

100 grams of roughly chopped baby kale

1 peeled cucumber, slice in half lengthwise, remove seed and cut into slices

1 tbsp. of sesame seeds

For the dressing:

2 tsp of soy sauce

1 tsp of clear honey

Juice of 1 lime

1 tsp of sesame oil

1 tbsp. of extra virgin olive oil

Directions:

1. Clean your frying pan well and make sure it's dry, toast the sesame seeds for 2 minutes in the pan until fragrant and lightly browned. Set aside in a plate to cool.

2. To Make the Dressing

3. In a small cup, combine the lime juice, soy sauce, olive oil, sesame oil and honey together.

4. Place the kale, cucumber, parsley, red onion and bok choy in a large bowl and mix gently. Pour dressing over salad and mix together.

5. Serve the salad in two different plates and add shredded chicken on top. Just before serving, sprinkle with sesame seeds.

Nutrition: kcal: 304 fat 6 protein 33 carbs 35

CPSIA information can be obtained
at www.ICGtesting.com
Printed in the USA
BVHW011016150321
602551BV00001B/87